The Little Book of Health for

Women

Your body – your life

Sharon Platt-McDonald
MScRHV RM RGN

First published 2010

© 2010 The Stanborough Press Ltd

British Library Cataloguing in Publication Data.
A catalogue record for this book is available from the
British Library.

ISBN 1-904685-86-2

Published by The Stanborough Press Ltd,
Grantham, Lincolnshire.

Designed by Abigail Murphy

Printed in Thailand.

Introduction

As women we juggle so many roles, agendas and expectations that sometimes we neglect our own needs. Here we offer a moment of peace to come away from it all and reflect on caring for *you*. This book reviews some of the key health issues which impact women's physical and emotional wellbeing and gives some guidance on how best to preserve your health.

There are two sections. The first includes sound bites on health research, with quick tips and health nuggets on a range of topical issues. Section two takes a more detailed look at some key health challenges.

Try to make your health needs a high priority. If you are already doing so, keep going, as this will pay dividends in the future. If not, I hope you will embrace the tips and advice to enhance your health and wellbeing. *You are worth it!*

Sharon

1. Physical wellbeing
Physical activity

Research undertaken by the Women's Sport and Fitness Foundation estimates that an alarming 80% of women are not doing enough exercise.

Being active as we age is crucial to our wellbeing, especially as some people tend to gain weight with age.

Quick activity tips for women at work

Even during your work schedule there are some simple movements which will increase your levels of physical activity.

• Phone calls. When you are on the phone, instead of sitting, stand up. Standing increases the metabolic rate slightly, so it's good to break up long periods of sitting. Standing also encourages you to move more, as you tend to pace while talking on the phone.

• Email versus direct contact. Rather than sitting in your chair and sending an email to your colleague in another department, walk down the hallway for direct communication and gain some vital movement. While in the office, maintain as much activity as possible.

Quick activity tips to do at home

• Increase the pace when hoovering to burn a few more calories and get the job done more quickly!

• Instead of using the dishwasher, wash and dry the dishes by hand as this acts as a mini hand-and-arm workout.

• While watching TV, raise and lower your legs. This helps the circulation, assists in toning and keeps lower limbs supple.

Physical activity while on the move

•While walking try increasing your pace, as brisk walking burns more calories.

• During a train or bus journey, standing is a good idea. Instead of holding on tightly, loosen your grip and allow your body to relax. This enables you to depend on your sense of balance and strengthens your core balance.

Physical activity as you age

German researchers found that exercise during the menopause is especially crucial and can reduce the risk of breast cancer. They discovered that physical activity affects hormonal processes in the body, which has a significant impact on reducing cancer risks.

Further studies indicate that even after the menopause the benefits of exercise continue to be pronounced. Professor Karen Steindorf reports: 'It might be gardening, cycling or walking to the shops. Our advice to women is to stay or become physically active in the second half of your life. You will not only reduce your risk of cancer, but also benefit your bones, heart and brain.'

A Japanese study followed over 30,000 women aged 40-69 to test the value of exercise as they aged. It found that women who walked for an hour or more a day and included additional weekly exercise of up to an hour reduced their risk of developing breast cancer by more than half. The results were the same for women who were post-menopausal, which proves that it's never too late to get moving!

Sharing the message

Passing on the message of increased activity is key advice even for young females. Studies now show that exercise in the teenage years is linked to bone health in older years. In a recent Japanese study, researchers asked post-menopausal women about the exercise they undertook in adolescence. It was found that those who exercised more as teenagers had better bone health as adults. The study concluded that playing weight-bearing sports like netball during teenage years can make the bones stronger even forty years later.

Nutritional wellbeing

Food that harms

- **Red meat**. A recent University of Leeds study found that eating red meat could significantly increase the chance of post-menopausal women developing breast cancer. Older women who ate a 2oz portion of red meat every day had a 56% greater risk of breast cancer compared to women who ate none. Red meat is high in saturated fat, which elevates cholesterol levels and affects oestrogen production. Previous research found that this oestrogen link has been indicative of a higher rate of breast cancer.

- Numerous studies have also linked high red meat consumption with increased risk of bowel cancer. As a result of these findings Cancer Research UK advises people to eat smaller and fewer portions of red meat and processed meat and instead to try pulses or beans as substitutes.

Food that heals

• **Flaxseed.** Findings published in the *Journal of the Society for Integrated Oncology* showed that in post-menopausal women who did not take HRT, flaxseed could decrease hot flushes. Women who took flaxseed (40g daily) as a therapeutic intervention for six weeks noticed a decrease of up to 57% in the severity and frequency of hot flushes. They also reported improvements in other symptoms such as brighter mood, less joint and muscle pain and alleviation of chills.

Foods for females

• **Beans and lentils** – Low in fat, calories and sodium but high in fibre. Important for people with diabetes due to their low glycaemic index (sugar in carbohydrates).

• **Blueberries** – Rich in antioxidants which help to prevent premature ageing.

- **Curry** – Antioxidants found in curry may help break up plaques in the brain that cause Alzheimer's disease.

- **Garlic** – Researchers are looking at its antioxidant effects and anti-ageing benefits. Garlic contains allicin which encourages the elimination of cholesterol from the body. It's also known for its immune-boosting properties.

- **Kiwi** – High in vitamin C and antioxidants, good for skin, bones and teeth.

- **Oatmeal** – Eaten daily, it can lower cholesterol levels. Good fibre and protein content help to keep you feeling full and avoid snacking.

- **Pistachios** – High in vitamin B6 and copper to increase energy. May also raise levels of good cholesterol (HDL).

- **Soya** – Beneficial post-menopause and thought to be cancer protective for older women.

- **Spinach** – Rich in nutrients and antioxidants. Contains lutein, essential for eye health. Also a good source of vitamins B, C and E, potassium, calcium, iron, magnesium and omega-3 fatty acids.

- **Sprouts** – Packed with fibre and immune-boosting vitamins C and A.

- **Sweet potatoes** – Rich in beta-carotene, an antioxidant that fights ageing.

- **Tomatoes** – Full of lycopene, believed to help lower cancer risks, heart disease and macular degeneration (ageing eye disease).

- **Walnuts** – Eaten daily will provide nutrients like omega-3 fatty acids and vitamin E, good for heart, brain and skin health.

Healthy food treats

Eating healthily doesn't rule out giving yourself the occasional treat. Try the following tasty snacks/desserts.

- Berries with frozen yoghurt.

- Cut bananas into slices and freeze them.

- Instead of fattening ice-cream, try making a plant-based alternative in an ice-cream maker by using a blend of bananas and mangoes with a little soya milk sweetened with honey.

Immune building

As women leading busy lives we experience
the tension between domestic and career
obligations. We juggle the many responsibilities
of being daughter, wife, mother, grandmother,
and sometimes the multi-tasking takes its toll.
Our immune system can come under strain.

Quick immune building juices:

• 3 large carrots, 3 sticks of celery, 1 beetroot, 3 cloves of garlic, a sprig of parsley (juiced).

• 1 banana, 1 apple, 1 beetroot, wheatgrass powder and spirulina – drink at breakfast time.

Cardiovascular health

One in six women and one in five men die
of coronary heart disease in the UK, making it
the number one killer.

Research from the *European Heart Journal*
reveals that women with high blood pressure
have an increased risk of cardiovascular and
other diseases, being up to three times more
likely to develop diabetes than those with low
blood pressure.

Studies have identified that co-enzyme Q10 supplements can help to lower blood pressure.

Daily exercise, a low-salt, low-fat diet and good stress management programmes have also helped to reduce the risk of cardiovascular illnesses.

Cancer facts

- Melanoma, the most deadly form of skin cancer, is now the leading cancer in young British women.

- Breast cancer is currently the most common form of cancer in the UK and the leading cause of cancer deaths in women. It is also the primary cause of deaths among black women over 30. Worldwide, over a million women are diagnosed with breast cancer every year.

- Bowel cancer is the second most common cancer in women.

• Cervical cancer is the second most common cancer in females under 35 in the UK.

• Lung cancer registers as the third most common form of cancer in women. More than 16,600 women were diagnosed with lung cancer in the UK in 2006.

• Cancer of the uterus is the fourth most common cancer in women in the UK, with 6,891 cases diagnosed in 2005.

• Ovarian cancer is the fifth most common cancer, most prevalent in women who have never had children.

More than 14,000 British women are diagnosed with gynaecological cancers each year.

Cancer Research UK

Global incidence of breast cancer

(Per 100,000 population, 2002 estimates)

Country	Incidence	Mortality
China	18.7	5.5
Zimbabwe	19	14.1
India	19.1	10.4
Brazil	46	14.1
Singapore	48.7	15.8
Italy	74.4	18.9
Netherlands	86.7	27.5
UK	87.2	24.3
Denmark	88.7	27.8
France	91.9	21.5
USA	101.1	19

Source: GLOBOCAN 2002

Factors in reducing cancer risk

Studies have indicated that the onset of cancer is mostly related to lifestyle factors and have suggested the following to reduce its occurrence.

- Vegetarian or mostly plant-based diet

- Non-smoking history

- Non-drinker

- Daily physical activity or exercise most days a week for a minimum of 30 minutes

- Ideal body weight

- Avoidance of sunburn

- Reducing exposure to toxins

- Good stress management

- Adequate rest and sleep

Sexual health

The charity Wellbeing of Women (WoW) estimates that over half of the women in the UK experience problems with their reproductive organs at some time. The list of complaints includes everything from premenstrual tension (PMS) to cervical cancer.

Many women suffer 'female' problems in silence, either because they feel embarrassed to speak to their GP or they are worried about the outcome. WoW has produced a booklet: *What Every Woman Should Know About Her Body* in order to help women better understand their health and give them confidence to seek help.

For more information email
wellbeingofwomen@rcog.org.uk

Key health examinations

Clinical breast examination: This is a physical examination in which a doctor or other healthcare professional checks the breasts and underarms for lumps or other changes that could be signs of breast cancer. Regular self-examination is also encouraged.

Mammogram: This is a special X-ray of the breast that often reveals cancers too small to feel. A woman's risk of breast cancer increases with age. Women aged 50 to 70 in the UK are invited for breast screening every three years.

Smear test: This is undertaken by a practice nurse, doctor or gynaecologist. Cells from the cervix and vagina are gently scraped, sent for analysis and checked for signs of abnormality. In the UK women between the ages of 25-49 are invited for smear tests every three years and women 50-65 every five years.

Pelvic examination: This is usually undertaken by a doctor who checks the uterus, vagina, ovaries and rectum for any changes in shape or size. An instrument called a spectrum is used to widen the vagina canal so that the upper part of the vagina and the cervix can be examined.

Menstruation

The time-of-the-month can be challenging for many women. Around 30% in the UK suffer from menorrhagia (heavy menstrual flow) or dysmenorrhoea (painful periods). Here are some helpful tips.

• **Take phytoestrogens**. These plant-based chemicals act like hormones and affect the production of oestrogen, helping to balance it. Phytoestrogens are present in chickpeas, lentils and tofu.

• **Include omega-3 oils**. These oils produce hormone-like substances called prostaglandins which help to control blood flow.

• **Increase iron intake.** More iron is needed to keep the blood healthy and prevent anaemia if periods are heavy. Good sources are leafy green vegetables and dried fruits. One teaspoon of black strap molasses in warm water morning and evening also helps. Vitamin C helps the body process iron, so include orange juice or oranges in your daily diet. If iron count remains low a supplement may be necessary.

• **Ensure sufficient vitamin A.** This is essential for the healthy growth of body cells, including red blood cells, and is closely associated with hormone levels. Excessive bleeding and longer periods (6+ days) can affect vitamin A levels. Vitamin A is found in green and yellow vegetables and fruit (spinach, carrots, pumpkin, mango, papaya).

• **Exercise regularly.** Exercise can improve period pain and alleviate stress. Ensure you exercise regularly or engage in physical activity 5-6 times a week for at least 30 minutes.

• **Monitor weight.** Research shows that there is a correlation between higher body fat and higher levels of oestrogen. In people who are overweight the lining of the womb is also thicker. Both these factors can adversely affect menstruation. Assess your daily diet and exercise routine to reduce calories and keep weight within the ideal range.

Premenstral syndrome (PMS)

Premenstrual syndrome (PMS) involves a variety of physical, mental and behavioural symptoms related to the menstrual cycle. Symptoms usually occur during the days before the period commences and cease after the first few days of flow. It is estimated that up to 80% of women experience symptoms. This can affect mood, eating, sleeping and working routine. The key factor causing PMS appears to be hormonal changes. (Up to 8% of women may have a more severe condition called premenstrual dysphoric disorder [PMDD], now classified as a mental health disorder.)

Tips for dealing with PMS

- **Exercise** increases circulation, reduces stress hormones, raises energy levels, enhances mood and general wellbeing.

- **Avoid junk foods.** These are generally poor in nutrients. Choose foods rich in calcium. Cut back on sugar and fat.

- **Fibre.** Increase consumption of fibre. Eat complex carbohydrates – whole-grain breads, pasta and cereals.

- **Avoid salt**, particularly near to your period, to reduce bloating and fluid retention.

- **Avoid caffeine** intake to feel less tense and irritable.

- **Avoid alcoholic beverages** which can make you feel more depressed.

- **Practise deep-breathing exercises** to help reduce headaches, anxiety or trouble with sleeping.

- **Ensure adequate sleep** – about 8 hours a night.

Polycystic ovary syndrome (PCOS)

Affecting approximately 5% of women (of all races), PCOS is an endocrine disorder. It is reported to be the most common hormonal disorder among women of reproductive age and is a leading cause of infertility.

The symptoms and severity differ greatly. The most common symptoms are: an excessive amount of male hormones (androgens), irregular menstruation (anovulation) and obesity. The causes of PCOS are unknown, but there are strong correlations between insulin resistance, diabetes and obesity and the onset of PCOS.

Tips

- **Exercise** is essential for managing PCOS, particularly for women who are overweight. Thirty minutes is advised.

- **Monitor weight.** Losing weight can improve symptoms like high blood pressure.

- **Stress less.** To reduce stress and help balance mood, relaxation sessions are a good idea. Light stretching exercises encourage muscle relaxation and are good for toning.

- **Eat wholesome foods.** Go for foods with a low glycaemic index (GI) that do not cause a surge in blood sugar levels or result in high output of insulin to cope with raised blood sugars.

Sexual intimacy – health benefit

The University of Pennsylvania and Stanford University undertook a series of studies investigating sexuality in women. The researchers found several health benefits in women who engaged in regular sexual intercourse within a loving, committed relationship. The impact on physical and emotional wellbeing was found to be as follows:

- Increased fertility
- Regular menstrual cycle
- Shorter menses
- Increased oestrogen levels
- Delayed menopause
- Delayed ageing
- Enhanced brain activity
- Improved memory

Recent scientific reports have revealed brain imaging studies which show that decreased levels of oestrogen are associated with general decreased brain activity and poor memory. When oestrogen levels were enhanced through regular sexual activity (at least once a week) it was found to enhance overall brain activity as well as improve memory.

Numerous studies on human sexuality have demonstrated that intimacy and emotional bonding are perhaps the most important factors in creating a positive and healthy sexual experience.

Sexual abuse and sexual violence against women

Women who have experienced this area of trauma usually have significant challenges in regards to their emotional and physical attitude towards sexual intimacy. However, counselling and therapy have been shown to enhance recovery and encourage healing to enjoy a healthy sexual relationship.

Reproduction

A study found the following facts in regard to the reproductive age range for women.

- 75% of women aged 30 trying to conceive will become pregnant within 1 year.

- 66% of women at 35 aiming for pregnancy will succeed within a year.

- 44% of women aged 40 trying to conceive will be successful within 1 year.

Tips to aid reproduction

• **Take folic acid** from the time you commence trying to conceive. This should be continued until the end of the first 12 weeks of pregnancy to prevent neural tube defects in your baby such as spina bifida.

• **Exercise** to improve mood and energy levels as well as to get in optimal shape. Fitness before pregnancy helps to ensure you keep active during pregnancy.

- **Eat wholesome foods.** This will ensure you have the correct nutrients to sustain a pregnancy and nourish your baby. Fast foods and processed foods should be limited or avoided if possible. Increase your intake of fruit and vegetables.

- **Don't smoke** and avoid passive smoking. Research proves that mothers who smoke are at higher risk of miscarriage. Babies of mothers who smoke are more likely to have lower birth weights. The advice not to smoke applies to your spouse as the quality of sperm is affected by cigarettes as well as illegal drugs and alcohol.

Pregnancy facts

- **Supplements.** In a report from the *British Journal of Obstetrics and Gynaecology* researchers suggest that calcium supplements may help women reduce their risk of pre-eclampsia and high blood pressure during pregnancy.

- **Folic acid** is vital for pregnant women and for the development of a healthy foetus. This B vitamin helps the body to make healthy new cells. Studies show that women on the pill may have depleted levels of this vitamin. Asparagus and kale have a high folic acid content – good news for vegetarian mums-to-be.

- **Low magnesium** is often associated with repeated miscarriage in women.

- **Keep fit.** One safe way to exercise is aqua aerobics. A study in the journal *Reproductive Health* researched two groups of low-risk pregnant women. One group did no exercise during their pregnancy and the other undertook moderate exercise three times a week doing water aerobics. The women in both groups were followed up during labour. It was found that just over a quarter of the women in the exercise group requested pain relief during labour in comparison with 65% of those who did no exercise.

• **Music therapy.** Research reveals that the tempo of music can be health enhancing for pregnant women. Music with a tempo close to the human heartbeat could help with relaxation. In a study published by the *Journal of Clinical Nursing*, pregnant women who listened to particularly soothing sounds like classical music, lullabies and nature sounds for thirty minutes each day for two weeks experienced significantly less stress, anxiety and depression than others who did not listen to this type of music.

Cystitis

A recent study by scientists in Massachusetts found that cranberries are effective in staving off cystitis. Cranberries appear to prevent e coli bacteria – the cause of cystitis and kidney infections through negatively impacting the renal organs (bladder, urethra and kidneys). Two glasses a day were found to be the most beneficial. Most supermarkets now stock cranberry juice so it is easily accessible.

Endocrine health

Many women in their 50s would admit that they felt tired, had weight concerns, suffered mood swings, some with regular low moods, and experienced restlessness and irritability on occasions.

Most put their symptoms down to the menopause. However, they are also symptoms of an under-active thyroid and could be hypothyroidism which is more common with ageing. Women are affected with thyroid disease at least 5-10 more times than men. All women should be tested by age 50 and younger if there is a family history of thyroid disease.

A significant percentage of younger women experience these symptoms, too, as part of their battle with premenstrual tension, so it is easy to see how an under-active thyroid gland can be missed if the symptoms are not recognised.

If you are experiencing these symptoms, it is important to seek advice promptly as symptoms can worsen and leave you feeling quite unwell. A visit to the GP will ensure that you receive a simple blood test.

Musculoskeletal health

Osteoporosis occurs when the bone mass becomes depleted, usually as a result of insufficient calcium. It is often called the 'silent disease' as it generally occurs without any symptoms and is not noticed until bone breakage results due to the weakness of the bone. Something as simple as a slight knock, sudden strain or fall can be enough to cause breakage of a bone.

Protective factor. The hormone oestrogen reduces the amount of bone broken down and so helps to protect against osteoporosis. The ovaries produce oestrogen from puberty until the menopause. After the menopause the lack of oestrogen can cause quicker breakdown of the bone.

Risk factors for osteoporosis:

If the number of years that a woman produces oestrogen is reduced, this may increase the risk of osteoporosis. This can be impacted by:

- early menopause (before the age of 45)

- total hysterectomy before the age of 45 (including removal of both ovaries)

- excessive exercising can reduce hormone levels, negatively impacting the menstrual cycle, and result in cessation of periods for a prolonged time

Other factors include:

- gender – women's bones are
  smaller than men's

- age – osteoporosis risk increases with age

- race – Caucasian or Asians are at greater
  risk than African-Caribbeans

- family history of osteoporosis – particularly
  a history of hip fracture in a parent

- very low body mass index (the combined measurement of weight and height)

- low levels of dietary calcium or vitamin D

- excessive alcohol consumption or smoking

- previous fragility fracture (bone fracture from a minor accident)

- long-term immobility (for example, confined to bed)

Some disorders, diseases and medicines can increase osteoporosis risk:

- rheumatoid arthritis

- over-active thyroid (disorders like hyperthyroidism)

- digestive disorders that affect nutrient absorption, such as Crohn's Disease, coeliac disease and chronic liver disease

- a disorder of calcium metabolism known as hyperparathyroidism

- bone disorder such as ankylosing spondylitis

- other conditions, such as kidney disease

- long-term use of steroids

- long-term use of heparin

- cancer medication like aromatase (used in the treatment of breast cancer in women)

Prevention

Medical experts state that osteoporosis is preventable. The following tips, mostly lifestyle changes, help ensure the maintenance of healthy bones.

• Take regular exercise as it aids the absorption of calcium and increases blood flow. Weight bearing exercises are good for strengthening the bone. Additionally, the National Osteoporosis Society recommends high impact exercise like jogging, aerobics, tennis, weight-training, dancing and brisk walking.

• Avoid smoking and alcohol as these can deplete calcium levels.

• Get the recommended daily intake of calcium (700mg) through a healthy diet. Although found in milk and dairy products such as cheese and yoghurt, plant-based sources of calcium are dried apricots or figs and some green leafy vegetables such as watercress and kale.

Skin care

One of the obvious signs of ageing is the reduction of elasticity of the skin and loss of muscle tone. This is one aspect of ageing that women often worry about, and countless 'remedies' have been produced.

If it wrinkles, crinkles, sags or bags, if it drops or droops, the pharmaceutical and cosmetic industries have 'cures' which smooth, firm and lift. Indeed, age-reversal is topical and it's big business.

However, studies show that certain vitamins and natural oils have been used effectively to maintain skin health as the body ages.

Vitamin aid

Research indicates that creams rich in vitamin C and E nourish and preserve skin due to their antioxidant properties which protect against cell degeneration.

Pamper time

Peppermint oil – good for cooling down and feels refreshing. Place a few drops in the bath and enjoy or inhale after putting a few drops on a tissue.

Lavender oil – good for aiding relaxation. Use in the bath for a lengthy soak. Rub a few drops into your feet for a gentle foot massage after a long day.

Starflower oil – has been found to nourish the skin and enhance its smoothness.

Jojoba oil – In its pure form, jojoba oil mimics the face's natural sebum and its non-greasy consistency means it's readily absorbed. It's reported to boost blood flow to the skin and absorb impurities. It is used as a facial cleanser as it is suitable for most skin types and helps to balance out the skin's moisture levels. It's a great healing oil when applied to sore, chapped lips. Equally excellent is its use for hair and general body skin care.

Vitamin E oil – Useful in the treatment of skin scars. Also good as an emollient for the skin.

Spiritual wellbeing

'Older women are more grateful to God than older men, and they receive greater stress-buffering health effects due to this gratitude,' states a recent report from the University of Florida in Gainesville and Wayne State University in Detroit. It was found that older adults, particularly women, use prayer more than any other alternative therapy for health. The results revealed 96% of participants using prayer specifically to cope with stress.

In numerous studies prayer and spirituality have been linked to:

- better overall health

- fewer cardiovascular diseases like hypertension

- less stress, even during difficult times

- less depression

- more positive feelings

- better psychological wellbeing

- greater ability to handle stress

Social wellbeing

Its official! Gossiping is good for women! (Friendly gossip, just to clarify.) According to a University of Michigan study, light-hearted talk among women is health enhancing. The benefits were:

• raised levels of the female hormone progesterone, which has a role in bonding

• stress reduction

• feelings of happiness

These results were ascertained after scientists monitored 160 pairs of women who were divided into two groups. One group was given emotional-type questions like: 'Who would be your ideal dinner guest?' The other group was given a paper on botany to proofread. After twenty minutes the 'gossip' group had progesterone levels that had either increased or remained the same. However the proofreading group had decreased levels of progesterone.

So, ladies, increase the chitchat to boost those progesterone levels and gain the health benefits!

2. An in-depth look
Emotional wellbeing
Stress – gender impact

Studies show equal numbers of women and men complaining of stress. However, they are stressed by different things and react in different ways.

Stressors for women

Poor work/life balance – Many working women carry the lion's share of childcare, housework and caring for older relatives.

Pregnancy – Stressor: Hormonal changes, pregnancy related symptoms, altered body image.

New baby – Stressor: lone parenting, relationship difficulties with partner, financial concerns, career break or change, postnatal depression.

Children – Stressor: high dependency. A parenting magazine survey found that 51% of full-time mothers felt regularly stressed, compared to 29% of working women without children.

Caring for relatives – Stressor: repetitive and demanding chores. Nearly seven million carers in Britain (mostly women) looking after disabled or frail elderly relatives.

Bereavement – Women are more likely to suffer bereavement as they generally live longer than men.

How women cope

Women are generally better than men at seeking help when stressed, and more comfortable sharing their feelings and talking about everyday life challenges. Twice as many women as men see their doctors about anxiety, depression and stress rather than waiting for a physical problem to develop.

Women often cope with several demands because they are naturally more 'multi-tasked'.

Reports indicate that both men and women benefit equally from effective stress management. Equally effective is good time management and better work-life balance to prevent overload. Other therapeutic interventions like massage, exercise, prayerful reflection, deep breathing, listening to relaxing music and so on have also been found to be beneficial.

Midlife crisis?

What is it?

Researcher Nancy Better defines midlife crisis as 'a time of profound psychological turbulence that usually occurs between the ages of 38 and 55, and often results in dramatic life changes. It can last from 2 to 12 years; the defining symptom is a sense that the values that have guided you for many years no longer hold meaning.'

Key symptoms

Frequently reported problems include:

- Irritability

- Lowered self-esteem

- Sudden change in sexual behaviour including loss of libido (sex drive) or increased sexual appetite

- Sudden change of image, particularly dressing much younger than one's age in an attempt to look 'youthful'

- Behavioural changes including secrecy, isolation

- Significant change in sleep pattern including insomnia or oversleeping

- Addictive behaviour, including significant increase in time spent watching TV, long periods engaged on the Internet

- Fatigue

- Loss of interest in work, family
  and usual circle of friends

- New circle of friends to the exclusion
  of former friendships

- Depression characterised by low moods and
  (often apparently unaccountable) feelings
  of sadness and lethargy

- Extramarital affair

Some have also reported the following symptoms:

- Muscle and joint stiffness

- Night sweats

- Dry skin

- Hair loss

- Weight gain

What causes it?

Unresolved negative experiences and emotions – difficult childhood experiences and traumatic relationships.

Working life insecurities – job changes, lack of promotion, redundancies, early retirement.

Health challenges – unexpected illnesses following prior good health.

Becoming a carer – caring for disabled or sick partners and relatives.

Fears about mortality – awareness of moving towards old age and inevitable death.

Empty nest syndrome – feelings of loss or emptiness as children leave home.

Marriage break-up – due to changes in perspectives, feelings and responsibilities.

Financial challenges – due to work changes in hours, loss of job or debt problems.

Gender differences

Nancy Better reports: 'My research shows that women's midlife crises are likely to stem from introspection, a family event, or problem, such as divorce or death or disappointment in their children. Men's midlife crises are more likely to be driven by work or career issues. Even though more women these days are working, I find that these differences haven't entirely disappeared. But men and women alike can be physically reckless, turning to adventure sports or extramarital affairs to deal with midlife angst.'

Studies show that women are thrust into midlife crisis because they reach a certain age and find they finally have the opportunity to do all the things they have put off doing while caring for their family.

• A woman's children are grown and suddenly she has the opportunity to do all those things she put off while being a mother.

- Both she and her husband have worked hard for several years. Now financially secure, she views this security as her opportunity to explore all those things she has put on the back burner.

- Additionally, as they go through the menopause women experience both biological and psychological changes which, if not managed effectively, can affect emotional wellbeing. The psychological changes a woman experiences can cause her to question her life up to that point and what possible changes she could now make.

Risk factors

Women have to come to terms with many physiological and social changes which have an impact on emotions and psychological wellbeing. At the same time there are competing priorities for them to undertake the roles of mother, wife, career woman and carer.

You may recognise some of the following behaviours and feelings in yourself or other females. Take some time to think about a positive response to each issue and, if necessary, how you can find the appropriate support to assist you.

What women experience

Psychological triggers

1. Changes in body image may affect confidence and self-esteem.

2. Husband may become interested in other women and she feels displaced.

3. Feeling that she is getting old, she processes this as a negative experience.

Physiological triggers

1. With the commencement of the menopause she encounters uncomfortable symptoms and no longer feels attractive.

2. Changes in hair, skin, weight or body shape may make her feel less feminine.

3. Lowered oestrogen levels cause both physiological and emotional changes in women.

Sociological triggers

1. Now past childbearing age she may feel 'redundant'.

2. Early retirement from work may make her feel as if she is no longer contributing to society.

The following tips have been
found to be beneficial:

• **Maintain good health habits**. Avoid the
temptation to use alcohol, nicotine or other
drugs as a means of release.

• **De-stressing treatments and exercises**.
Many complementary approaches, such
as hydrotherapy, massage and
aromatherapy, have been found to
have a powerful relaxing effect.

- **Exercise**. The effects of exercise in promoting positive moods and reducing mild depression are well-documented.

- **Prayer**. Having close friends and family pray for you during this time is key to maintaining your emotional and spiritual wellbeing. Trust and reliance on God can sustain you at this vulnerable time.

- **Acceptance**. Accept the fact that ageing is a natural process and we will all have to face it at some point.

• **Reassurance**. Life is a journey full of transitions. The journey from youth to middle age and into old age are transitions that may seem challenging and uncomfortable. Rather than being fearful of what may transpire, it can also be seen as an opportunity to re-evaluate and perhaps change the direction of life. Embrace a positive mindset which captures the belief that ageing is not simply about having to give things up, but about new ways of doing things.

Self-help/alternative treatments

• **Daily vitamin B complex** builds
the nervous system for those
experiencing nervous anxiety.

• **Christian counselling**. This encourages
expression and assists in addressing issues.

- **Regular exercise**. Good for maintaining holistic health. Releases endorphins also known as 'happy hormones' which elevate mood.

- **Healthy eating**. Research points to the more natural plant-based diet as being more beneficial to physical and mental health.

Depression

Depression rates in women are twice as high as in men. This is due in part to hormonal factors, more so in relation to premenstrual syndrome, commonly called PMS, premenstrual dysphoric disorder (PMDD), postpartum depression and perimenopausal depression.

Signs and symptoms – Women are more likely than men to experience pronounced feelings of guilt, sleep excessively, overeat and gain weight. Research also indicates that women are more likely to suffer from a condition called Seasonal Affective Disorder, known as SAD.

Risk factors for depression

- Family history of mood disorders

- Childhood history of physical or sexual abuse

- Personal past history of mood disorders, especially during early reproductive years

- Loss of a parent before age 10 years

- Use of oral contraceptives, in particular those with a higher level of progesterone

- Use of gonadotropin stimulants as part of infertility treatment

- Ongoing psychosocial stressors

- Loss of social support system

- Job changes involving loss of status

Common signs and symptoms of depression include:

• **Loss of interest in life activities** – Decreased interest in daily activities, no interest in or ability to enjoy social activities, hobbies or sexual intimacy.

• **Poor concentration** – Difficulty focusing, making decisions or remembering things (typically short-term memory).

• **Feelings of helplessness and hopelessness** – A mindset that sees only challenges. Having a bleak outlook which expresses the view that things will not get better and an inability to impact or improve the situation.

• **Altered sleep patterns** – Insomnia (difficulty getting to sleep or waking in the early hours). Oversleeping (also known as hypersomnia) may be another indicator.

• **Appetite or weight changes** – Increased or decreased appetite. Significant weight loss or weight gain – for example, a change of more than 5% of body weight in a month.

• **Loss of energy** – Constantly feeling fatigued and physically drained, no matter how much rest one gets. Finds it difficult to execute even the smallest tasks and takes a long time completing them.

• **Neurological and physical changes** – This may include nervousness, anxiety, irritability, worry and/or physical symptoms such as sluggishness, palpitations, headaches, cramps or aches and pains that do not ease with treatment.

• **Self-loathing.** This includes negative self-talk and highlights perceived faults and mistakes as major character flaws. Experiences strong feelings of worthlessness or guilt resulting in harsh criticism of self.

Responding to depression

Working with medication and therapy

Depending on the cause and severity of the
depression, medication may be prescribed.
Patients should be encouraged to note the
effects of the medication and report any side
effects (including suicidal thoughts) to their
practitioners so other treatment options,
alternative medication or therapy
can be considered.

Depression recovery programmes

Therapeutic interventions like Dr Neil Nedley's world-renowned depression recovery programme, delivered via books and workbook, DVD or residential setting, has helped thousands in their recovery from depression. More information on these programmes and resources can be accessed at *www.drnedley.com*.

Food factors

A change in eating may occur when individuals experience depression. Lack of appetite, overeating, comfort eating or craving junk food is common. Some essential vitamins and fatty acids are often found to be lacking in the diet and are sometimes recommended as supplements for managing the condition.

• Fatty acids make up 15% of the brain's weight. Deficiencies in these omega-3 fatty acids are thought to contribute to severe mental health challenges, including depression. Vegetarian sources: flax.

• B vitamins, particularly B6, B9 and B12, are believed to benefit people with depression. Vegetarian sources: B6 – bananas, nuts and seeds, potatoes, whole-grain cereals; B9 – asparagus, nuts, peas, whole grains, yeast; B12 – seaweed, yeast extract.

• Tryptophan is a naturally occurring amino acid used by the body to make serotonin (an important brain chemical, affecting mood). Rich sources include bananas and oats.

Exercise

In mild cases, exercise has been found to be as effective as antidepressant drugs in reducing symptoms. Exercise increases the levels of endorphins (also known as happy hormones) which makes you less sensitive to pain and engenders a 'feel good' factor. Exercise enhances health and wellbeing, improves physical appearance, boosts confidence and raises self-esteem. All these factors help to improve mood and fight depression. The challenge is the motivation to begin exercising or maintaining it. Gentle encouragement to commence a manageable programme is useful.

Dealing with the menopause

What is the menopause?

The word *menopause* is defined as the point when a woman naturally stops ovulating and menstruation ceases. Menopause occurs when a woman comes to the end of her reproductive life and the levels of oestrogen and progesterone drop.

What are the symptoms?

'Going through the change' is a common description of what happens to a woman in midlife. Some women go through the menopause without much discomfort and few obvious changes. However, many women are faced with the challenges of annoying symptoms that affect their physical, emotional and social wellbeing.

A range of symptoms have been reported by women. Among them are:

Physical

Hot flushes, heart palpitations, headaches, night sweats, breast tenderness, irregular periods, bloating, weight gain, muscle tension, sore joints, vaginal dryness, loss of libido, frequent urination, urinary tract infections, fatigue, sleeplessness.

Emotional/mental

Mood swings, difficulty in concentration, irritability, aggressiveness, anxiety, feelings of sadness, depression, memory lapses or loss, lack of motivation, tension.

Coping with the emotional changes

Emotional symptoms of menopause like irritability and feelings of sadness are the most common. Reports on the outcome of natural interventions have found that symptoms like these can be managed effectively through lifestyle changes. This includes effective stress management to reduce stress, learning ways to relax and how to boost emotional resilience.

Tips for managing fluctuating emotions:

• Maintain regular exercise and eat healthily as part of a daily routine.

• Engage in a creative outlet that fosters a sense of achievement.

• Avoid tranquillisers and alcohol.

• Stay connected with family and community.

• Nurture friendships.

• Seek regular calming interventions like massage, prayerful reflection, deep breathing, listening to relaxing music and so on.

Natural interventions during the menopause

Menopause is a natural process which occurs at the end of every woman's reproductive life. As such it should be treated as naturally as possible.

In order to remain healthy and feel better emotionally and physically, there are a number of steps women in menopause and post-menopause can take to enable them to continue to enjoy life.

The following have been found to be beneficial health practices:

• Maintaining a balanced diet. Nutritionists recommend whole grains, cold pressed oils, leafy vegetables and nuts to help keep the body healthy and potentially relieve hot flushes.

• Soya may also ease mild hot flushes. It is best to use a small amount of non-genetically-modified soya products that are not over processed. The natural preparations of tofu, miso and tempeh are better options than the processed soya products.

• Omega 6 and Omega 3. Studies suggests that these essential fatty acids can help regulate hormones and combat mood swings. Good sources are flaxseed, pumpkin seeds and safflower. Research demonstrates a strong link between hormonal balance in women and their emotional wellbeing.

• Vitamin B complex is key to a healthy nervous system. B vitamin levels are often depleted due to emotional stress related to menopause. Vitamin B helps the body to perform the proper metabolic functions and assists in decreasing irritability and fatigue.

- Calcium is required daily to help keep bones strong.

- Vitamin D also assists in the prevention of osteoporosis brought on by the menopause.

- Avoidance of stimulants like caffeine and alcohol and toxins like smoking.

- Avoidance of junk food, excess salt and sugar.

- Choose foods that are low in saturated fat and cholesterol.

- Keep active. Exercise releases endorphins which give a feel good factor. Engage in weight-bearing exercises daily for at least 30 minutes.

- Dress in natural fabric to keep skin cool.

- Reduce stress.

- Vaginal lubricants can help lubricate the vagina and make sexual intercourse more comfortable.

• Some herbal medicines and teas can relieve symptoms. However it is strongly advised that GPs and health professionals be made aware of all herbs and alternative treatments. In fact, it is best to inform them before taking complementary medicine/therapy. Helpful herbs are: Black Cohosh can relieve hot flushes and vaginal dryness, has a sedative and relaxing effect and can also relieve anxiety and irritability. Red clover and Agnus Castus can help to minimise the discomforts of menopause.

Controlling or finding relief from some of the physical symptoms helps to improve emotional and mental wellbeing.

Support

Menopausematters.co.uk is an independent, clinician-led website. It provides easily accessible, up-to-date, accurate information about the menopause, menopausal symptoms and treatment options, including Hormone Replacement Therapy (HRT) and alternative therapies, so that women and health professionals can make informed choices about menopause management.

Final words of advice

There are many facets to good health physically, emotionally, spiritually and socially. Here are a few suggestions to ensure a wholesome, balanced life.

- Take up regular health screening available in relation to your age.

- Exercise regularly to improve circulation, co-ordination and balance.

- Increase vegetable protein like beans and lentils in place of meat.

- Replace saturated fats with unsaturated fats.

- Include at least four servings of pulses in your diet weekly.

- Eat at least one tablespoon of nuts or seeds every day.

- Drink 2 litres of water daily to boost brain function and keep skin healthy.

- Manage stress effectively.

- Have a balanced life with adequate rest and sleep.

- Nurture faith and trust in God, have an active prayer life and keep a positive attitude to encourage good spiritual and mental health.

- Avoid exposure to toxins.

- Watch for any signs of bodily changes and seek medical assessment.

- Enjoy social interaction with family and friends.

- Be happy! Find one thing each day for which you are grateful and give thanks for it.

- Moisturise skin daily.

Conclusion

I hope you have found this book an informative read. Whether this information has inspired you to rediscover the path to health, reinforced your commitment to an already well-established one, or simply provided interesting food for thought, it was a joy to share with you a sample of some of the recent research and published studies on issues impacting female health.

I hope you have been encouraged to continue or commence putting your health needs on your daily agenda. If you model good health principles you can inspire other women to do the same. Additionally, as women leading a healthy lifestyle in your homes, you are sending the positive message to your family members that health matters. May you experience the best of health and the best of life. Enjoy the journey!

Good health!